30 Day Paleo Challenge

Lose up to 30lbs in 30 Days!

By

CASSIDY WILSON

Table of Contents

Introduction: 30 Days Later...

At first glance, the span of 30 days may not seem like much. But a lot can happen in 30 days' time. In fact, it is said that every 30 days our body's skin cells and even the tissue of our lungs have completely regenerated. This is really pretty incredible if you think about it, this means that we all have a new set of lungs every single month of our life! How much more then, can we expect to see a dynamic, metabolic impact upon our weight? A lot!

After 30 days of any diet your body is virtually reset and reprogrammed to the parameters of that diet. And when a strict 30-day regimen of the paleo diet are employed you can expect some rather rapid and remarkable results. And the results of the 30-day Paleo challenge you can trust, because the Paleo challenge actually goes back quite a long time. All the way back to the Paleolithic era to be exact!

The main premise of the diet is simply to eat like our Paleolithic ancestors are said to have eaten; chewing on nuts, seedlings, and a whole lot of fiber filled roughage, and a whole lot of meat. Many today may not realize it but our ancestors were in fact super carnivores. And mainstream science has established that part of the reason why our Paleolithic ancestors tended to be so trim was the fact that they cut the vast bulk of carbs out of their diet and mostly munched on meat.

This sort of diet plan is similar to the perhaps more famous diet of Dr. Atkins. Many ask what is the difference between the Atkins Diet and Paleo? The main difference is the kind of meat that the Atkins diet recommends as opposed to the meat that the Paleo Diet espouses. On Atkins dieters tend to eat a large amount of fat filled meat such as greasy pork products and other over processed foods that can be really bad for your vital organs in large quantities.

But Paleo on the other hand seeks to go back to nature and take the "process" out of food completely! You see, Paleo is not just some carb cutting gimmick it is an attempt to refine your entire lifestyle, and the Paleo Diet seeks to refine it in 30 days' time! By the end of your 30 days on Paleo you should feel rejuvenated and completely renewed. If you follow the regimen presented in this book you are hitting the reset button and making some critical changes to your own constitution that will last well after the first 30 days have passed.

Chapter 1: Getting Started on your Challenge

There can be no denying it, any time you set out to change a significant part of your routine it is a challenge. And that is very fitting for the 30-day Paleo Challenge, hence the name *challenge* is used in the title. In this chapter we will examine all of the nuances and idiosyncrasies for you to come out on your Paleo Challenge on top.

Buy the Right Produce

It may seem like a heavy dose of common sense that we are dishing out here, but there is no way that you can begin this challenge on proper footing unless you start off with the proper produce in the first place. There are certain things that you should have on your grocery list and also a few things that you should not. The first things that you should scratch off of that said list are anything containing a heavy dose of sugar, salt, or wheat based sorghum. These are just carb buildings nuisances so you should toss them at your earliest convenience.

You should also throw to the wayside much of your supply of heavily processed grain products. Unfortunately for most of us this means getting rid of about 90% of our pantry! We are a country that loves our processed foods plain and simple. But in order to be successful on this diet you will have to part with them! I can remember back to when I first tried the paleo challenge, and just how many of these over processed foods I had to ditch just to get started.

From the get go I had to empty out much of the contents of my cupboards and replace them with foods that were more paleo friendly. Instead of stockpiling heavily processed grains you should load up on some all-natural grass-fed meats such as lamb, chicken, goat, and beef. Animals that are strictly grass fed are free of the chemicals, hormones, and other toxins that make up most of the rest of our heavily processed and overtaxed food supply.

Grass fed meats also offer many other benefits such as more omega-3 fatty acids that aid in the reduction of heart disease and have even been shown to prevent cancer. It is for this reason that you see so many vitamins on store shelves touting that they are loaded to the max with "omega 4". But you don't have to pop pills to get this benefit folks, all you have to do is eat it! And the recipes in this book make full use of meat that came from these grass-fed animals, greatly bolstering your health in the process.

Along with grass fed meat from livestock animas, you should also get some cans of salmon, sardines, and tuna. You may have heard fish being referred to as a "brain food" and this is no accident. Fish are a crucial store of iodine. Iodine helps to regulate our thyroid gland as well as facilitate brain function. Our Paleolithic ancestors were dependent on fish for this very reason. Fish can help regulate neural function and with the endless variety of recipes available for the Paleo challenge, fish and fish products should not be overlooked.

Next to these meat staples you should also make sure that you have plenty of fruit packed up in your cupboards as well. But the veggies that you should avoid are those items full of starch such as potatoes, legumes, and lentils. People are surprised by this, but you should also nix any peanut consumption as well.

But interestingly, although you can't eat peanuts, peanut oil is a great part of the 30-Day Paleo Challenge. Along with sesame oil, olive oil, coconut oil, and a few others. These cooking oils are highly nutritious and should be on your list. You can find them at most department and health food stores. Buy the right produce folks!

Make a Food Calendar

While we aren't exactly tracking carbs, or counting calories during the 30-Day Paleo Challenge, we need to be mindful of the fact that we should have a general idea of what kinds of meals we are going to eat throughout the week. And this means creating what is called a "Food Calendar" a calendar in which you put your specific meal plans down on each calendar day of the week so that you can see them and know them without any difficulty. This is of great use in the 30-day Paleo Challenge. Just manage your routine and you can do the rest!

But if it is indeed a meal plan that you need to keep track of, you should move towards sectioning off your refrigerator and categorizing exactly what it is that you would like to eat. One of the easiest ways to do this is to demarcate on your calendar days; a time during the day for Breakfast, a time during the day for Lunch, and a time during the day for Dinner. Once you have these headings in place you can then put them down in real time on the calendar.

If you are a visual person like I am, having this daily reminder will help you out tremendously. And whatever it is that you plan out on your food calendar does not have to be set in stone either; this is just a template to get you started. You should make your list and check it twice, so you can make sure that you remain on task for the 30-day challenge from beginning to end.

Be Careful with Restaurants

Restaurants are the number one diet breaker known to man. And this is most especially the case with the Paleo diet. Since the Paleo diet requires you to eat some very specific foods and food combinations most restaurants will find it difficult to accommodate these demands. It is for this reason—if it is possible—I would recommend swearing off all restaurants until you successfully finish the 30-day paleo challenge.

But if you have no choice in the matter, and absolutely must eat out from time to time, I would recommend sticking to the rawest roughage that you can. This means very strict greens, and prime meat. It may take some specific bartering with the restaurant establishment but it can be done! They might ask you a lot of questions, and you just might find yourself on the spot

I can remember a time I went to a local steakhouse and had to order a specialty made salad because nothing else on the menu made sense. The waitress was nice enough, but it actually took two back and forth maneuvers between me, her, and the kitchen chefs to get it right! It took a little extra time but it was worth it since I was able to get through the evening without breaking my 30-day Paleo Challenge.

Chapter 2: Best Recipes for Your Paleo Breakfast

In order to be successful during any 30-day period, you will need to have a good morning meal to wake up to. You need to have the right balance of protein, vitamins and minerals to set you off on the right track. Our ancestors excelled on just a few morsels on that they foraged, and while we don't need to starve, our breakfasts should be similarly streamlined. We don't have to eat a nine-course meal in the morning, but a basic meal plan could do wonders.

Instead of just reaching for whatever's inside a store-bought box, we need to pay attention to what we are actually putting into our bodies. Unnecessary carbohydrates and over processed food should be avoided. So that means that sugary breakfast cereals are definitely out of the question. Trix may be for kids, but they aren't for the Paleo diet! Paleo emphasizes running the body on high performance food, and this means breaking that food down to its most essential elements.

Breakfast is the most important meal of the day, and all in all, it is a good meal for Paleo as well. Use this chapter to find an endless combination of ingredients and cooking methods to meet your needs when you first wake up. How you start your day usually dictates how you will end it, so let's start out on top! Check out all of these great breakfast recipes and decide which ones are best for you.

Vegetable Egg White Omelet

Egg whites are loaded with protein and other essential nutrients, and by avoiding the yolk you are avoiding excess cholesterol and fat. Admittedly our paleo ancestors didn't take the time to separate egg whites from egg yolks, but it is more than worth the effort if you do so. The Vegetable Egg White Omelet is as good for you as it tastes. Early in the morning nothing can beat this veggie omelet masterpiece!

Here are the exact ingredients:

2 egg whites

½ cup of water

¼ cup of vegetable oil

¼ cup of chopped onion

¼ cup of chopped red bell pepper

¼ cup of chopped green bell pepper

¼ cup of chopped carrots

First off, take your ½ cup of water and your 2 egg whites and beat them together in a medium sized mixing bowl. Now get out a small pan and add ¼ cup of vegetable oil, your ¼ cup of chopped onion, and set the burner on high. Stir the onions into the pan as it cooks for just a minute or two. Now add your ¼ cup of chopped red bell pepper, your ¼ cup of chopped green bell pepper, and your ¼ cup of chopped carrots.

Stir into the pan, and after a couple of minutes remove the veggies to a separate container. Now add your water/egg white mixture to the pan and put the burner on low heat. Lift the egg mixture with a spatula periodically so that it forms well and doesn't stick to the pan. After just a couple of minutes the egg should be thoroughly cooked. Now you can add your veggies on top of the eggs and fold the omelet over. Your Vegetable Egg White Omelet is ready to go!

Chili and Garlic Mushrooms

If you would like a little bit of spice in your breakfast life, check out this Chili and Garlic Mushrooms recipe! It comes fully loaded with mushrooms, garlic, olive oil, and just a hint of paprika! All in all, creating an irresistible blend for your morning routine! Paleo man didn't even know what he was missing with this one! Forget about coffee! As soon as I smell this combo cooking on the stove I shake off my sleepiness and wake right up! And you will too!

Here are the exact ingredients:

1 cup of button mushrooms

½ cup of chopped garlic

¼ cup of olive oil

¼ cup of ground paprika

To get started, put your ½ cup of chopped garlic, and your ¼ cup of ground paprika, into a medium sized mixing bowl and stir these ingredients together. Now deposit your cup of button mushrooms into the mix, followed by your ¼ cup of olive oil. Make sure you drizzle your ¼ cup of olive oil over the entire mixture.

Stir all of these ingredients together well. Now dump the contents of your bowl into a small pan, and set your burner on high. Stir the ingredients into the pan as they cook over the course of the next 10 minutes. Turn your burner off and allow the contents to cool off. Your Chili and garlic Mushrooms are prepared. Serve when ready.

Paleo Ham and Egg Breakfast cups

Here's a tasty paleo breakfast made right into a muffin breakfast up! While other diets might leave your body with a muffin top, with paleo you can rest assured that the only muffin tops you have to deal with are the ones you can eat! Ham and eggs have never been better!

Here are the exact ingredients:

1 cup of chopped ham

1 cup of chopped onion

1 cup of feta cheese

5 eggs

First, set your oven to 400 degrees. Now take out a muffin tin and place a paper muffin cup in each space of the tin. Get out a medium sized mixing bowl and crack your 5 eggs inside of it. Now add your cup of chopped ham, followed by your cup of chopped onion. Stir these ingredients together well and then pour them into your muffin cups in the muffin tin.

Make sure that each muffin cup is evenly filled with the ingredients. Once all the compartments of the tin are sufficiently filled, place the muffin tin into the oven and allow it to cook over the next 10 to 15 minutes. Once the ingredients are finished cooking, turn off your oven and take out your tin to cool. While cooling sprinkle your ½ cup of feta cheese on top of each muffin and serve

Raisin Omelet

Raisins are a lot better for us than most realize. And when these dried and shriveled up former grapes are coupled with the protein power of eggs, it's an unbeatable combination. The raisins really bring out the flavor of the eggs, and the eggs bring out the flavor of the raisins. Go ahead and have this morning powerhouse, and find out about it for yourself!

Here are the exact ingredients:

1 cup of raisins

3 eggs

¼ cup of cinnamon

¼ cup of all spice

¼ cup of nutmeg

Raisins really bring out the flavor of this omelet and it is the raisins that make up the first major step of this recipe. Put your cup of raisins in a saucepan, followed by your cup of water and set your burner on high. Let the raisins boil under the heat for a couple of minutes. Turn the burner off, and drain the water from your pan.

Now get out a mixing bowl and add your 3 eggs, ¼ cup of cinnamon, ¼ cup of all spice, and your ¼ cup of nutmeg. Mix all of these ingredients together. Pour your mixed ingredients on top of your raisins in the saucepan, covering them thoroughly. Now set your burner on medium heat and stir the ingredients into the pan as they cook. They should be stirred into one uniform paste.

After about just 1 or 2 minutes turn your burner off and allow the egg mixture to solidify into its omelet shape. After it stands for about 10 minutes flip the saucepan over a large plate and your raisin omelet—fully formed—should drop right out. Allow to cool at room temperature for a few minutes before serving. Enjoy your Raisin Omelet!

Scrambled Eggplant Breakfast

Tired of scrambled eggs? Then try scrambled eggplant! Freshly chopped eggplant, fried in olive oil and garnished with garlic, red bell pepper and onions. Nutritious and every bit as delicious, this Scrambled Eggplant Breakfast has everything you need to start your day off on a good note!

Here are the exact ingredients:

2 cups of chopped eggplant

½ cup of olive oil

1 cup of chopped onion

½ cup of chopped garlic

½ cup of chopped red bell pepper

¼ cup of turmeric

¼ cup of black pepper

¼ cup of basil

¼ cup of salt

Take your cup of chopped eggplant and dump it out onto a cutting board or other (clean) flat surface and then proceed to flatten it out and remove as much moisture as possible from it. Next, go to your stove and put a large frying pan on high heat and add your ½ cup of olive oil to the pan. Add your cup of chopped onions to the pan, followed by your ½ cup of red bell pepper and ½ cup of chopped garlic.

Proceed to stir these ingredients into the pan over the course of the next 10 to 15 minutes. Now go back to your flattened out and drained eggplant and begin crumbling it with your (clean) hands over the frying pan, letting it fall in small pieces over the ingredients. Once all of your eggplant is in place stir and cook the whole contents of your pan for another 5 minutes. Allow to cool and serve.

Scrambled Egg Stuffed Cucumber

This dish is great for the taste buds and great for your health as well! Scrumptiously scrambled eggs stuffed into a crisp cucumber shell! Every bite sends a crunch of delight straight to the brain!

Here are the exact ingredients:

1 large cucumber

2 eggs

This recipe is pretty straightforward. Crack your 2 eggs over a frying pan and scramble them over medium heat. Take your large cucumber, core out the center of it, and then deposit your scrambled eggs inside. Heat the whole thing up in a microwave for 20 seconds to ensure warmth, and enjoy!

Lemon Paleo Pancakes

Do you feel you need a real boost to get going in the morning? Well then—try some Lemon Paleo Pancakes to start your day off right! These pancakes pack a real punch and will have you back for seconds in no time flat.

Here are the exact ingredients:

¼ cup of apple sauce

1/2 cup of lemon juice

¼ cup of almond butter

¼ cup of coconut oil

2 eggs

In a small mixing bowl add your ¼ cup of apple sauce, ¼ cup of lemon juice, ¼ cup of almond butter and your 2 eggs. Stir all of these ingredients together well. Now get out a medium sized frying pan and put it on a burner set to low heat. Add your ¼ cup of coconut oil to this pan.

Let this heat up for a moment before adding your egg mixture to the pan as well. Stir this together briefly and then add your ½ cup of flour. Now stir all of these ingredients together and allow them to cook for a couple of minutes on each side. Get ready for some great Lemon Paleo Pancakes!

Veggie Fried Breakfast Fritters

If you are from the South you are probably familiar with this one! Fried Fritters have been a southern breakfast staple for a long time, but if they are arranged just right they can fit into a Paleo Diet quite well! Check out this recipe and find out for yourself just how tasty these Veggie Fried Breakfast Fritters really are!

Here are the exact ingredients:

½ cup of chopped sweet potatoes

½ cup of chopped carrot

½ cup of chopped zucchini

¼ cup of green peas

¼ cup of almond meal

¼ cup of coconut oil

¼ cup of salt

2 eggs

Get out a mixing bowl and add your ½ cup of chopped sweet potatoes, your ½ cup of chopped carrot, your ½ cup of chopped zucchini, your ¼ cup of green peas, your ¼ cup of almond meal, your ¼ cup of salt, and your 2 eggs to the bowl. Stir them together as well as you can. Once these ingredients are mixed together well, set the bowl to the side and allow them to settle in place for a few moments.

Now go to your stove and place a frying pan on high heat before adding your ½ cup of coconut oil to the pan. Make sure the oil evenly coats the entire pan. Now go back to your mixing bowl and with (clean) hands shape your ingredients into palm sized patties and place them down into the oil in your pan. You should be able to make about 3 patties. Serve when ready.

Bacon and Eggs

Here is a classic that no one ever gets tired of! But there is nothing more paleo than just plain old Bacon and Eggs! Exemplifying one of the great things about the Paleo diet, this meal allows you to have your fill of bacon right along with a healthy helping of eggs and all the paleolithic fixings!

Here are the exact ingredients:

1 cup of chopped bacon

½ cup of egg whites

¼ cup of pepper

1 cup of water

Place a medium sized saucepan on a burner set to high heat and add your cup of water to the pan. Now add your cup of bacon, your ½ cup of egg whites, and your ¼ cup of pepper. Set your burner for medium heat and stir the contents of the pan together while they cook. And after about 5 minutes your Bacon and Eggs are ready to eat!

Paleo Jicama Hash Browns

A great breakfast straight out of the Paleolithic Era! Although potatoes are usually avoided, with Jicama you can make some pretty sound hash browns. The secret ingredient here is actually the bacon fat (yes bacon fat). Because despite what you may have heard, having some forms of fat in your diet is actually good for you!

In fact, your body wouldn't be able to properly function without it! Studies have shown that fat improves brain function, helps regulate hormones and even helps to stave off the ravages of dementia! So, don't be shy with your bacon fat when you make this great blend of Paleo Jicama Hash Browns!

Here are the exact ingredients:

1 cup of shredded jicama

½ cup of bacon fat

¼ cup of pepper

Put your ½ cup of bacon fat into a medium sized frying pan, and set your burner on medium-high heat. Now add your cup of shredded jicama to a medium sized mixing bowl. Drizzle your ¼ cup of olive oil over the jicama. Take your (clean) hands and use them to shape the shredded jicama into rectangle shaped patties. Place these patties into your frying pan of bacon fat. Let the hash brown patties cook for about 2 or 3 minutes on each side. Serve when ready.

Chapter 3: Lunchtime Recipes with Paleo

Lunch is a great time to recharge our batteries and we need that extra boost of nutrition to help get us through our day. This is a difficult time for many of us who live our lives on the guy, and the lunch rush hour may bring on the temptation of quick fixes and fast food. But if you are tempted to go to the drive through or—even worse—reach for the vending machine, you need to read this chapter.

Here you will find some of the great alternatives you can make and possibly prep in advance for your lunch hour, so you don't have to settle for less. Take note of them and start putting them to practice. This chapter highlights some of the best lunch recipes to help you get through your 30-day paleo challenge!

Paleolithic Chicken Salad

This is a tasty paleolithic treat to get you through your midday routine! With juicy and satisfying shredded chicken breast generously marinated in mayonnaise, pesto, garlic, and basil, this dish provides just the kick your lunch hour needs! Pack up a batch of this Paleolithic Chicken Salad your next lunch break!

Here are the exact ingredients:

1 cup of shredded chicken breast

¼ cup of mayonnaise

½ cup of pesto

¼ cup of chopped garlic

½ cup of chopped basil

½ cup of chopped eggplant

1 cup of chopped tomatoes

½ cup of chopped avocado

½ cup of chopped black olives

Take out your chicken breast and put it in a medium sized sauce pan. Now add your cup of water to the pan and set your burner to high heat. Now get out a medium sized mixing bowl and add your ¼ cup of mayonnaise, your ½ cup of pesto, your ¼ cup of chopped garlic, your ½ cup of chopped basil, your 1 cup of chopped eggplant, and your cup of chopped tomatoes.

Mix these ingredients before adding your ½ cup of chopped avocado, and your ½ cup of chopped black olives. Stir these ingredients together well and add it to your shredded chicken breast in the pan. Stir vigorously for about 5 minutes as it cooks and then turn your burner off. This Paleolithic Chicken Salad is now ready for lunch!

Oven Roasted Okra

Okra is a great resource and one that our Paleolithic ancestors loved. These veggies were often roasted over the campfires of these cavemen and they can still be enjoyed in much the same way today! You may not have to forage for your Okra but a trip to your local grocer or health food store can be just as rewarding! Check out this amazing recipe for Oven Roasted Okra!

Here are the exact ingredients:

1 cup of chopped okra

¼ cup of coconut oil

¼ cup of salt

¼ cup of pepper

Go to your oven and set the temperature to 400 degrees. Now get out a cooking sheet and cover it with aluminum foil. Now place your okra on top of the foil covered cooking sheet. Drizzle the okra with your ¼ cup of coconut oil. Then take your ¼ cup of salt, and your ¼ cup of pepper and sprinkle it evenly over the okra. Place into the oven and allow it to cook for about 25 to 30 minutes. Turn off oven, allow these veggies to cool, and serve!

Lettuce Turkey Wraps

Fresh ground turkey cooked to perfection, garnished with garlic, onion, and ginger, and wrapped up in crunchy lettuce. You won't be able to get enough of this paleo dish. These turkey wraps are the best!

Here are the exact ingredients:

¼ cup of olive oil

½ cup of chopped garlic

½ cup of chopped onion

½ cup of ground turkey

¼ cup of cilantro

¼ cup of lime juice

¼ cup of ginger

3 leaves of lettuce

Add your ¼ cup of olive oil to a medium sized saucepan and place it on a burner set to high heat. Now add your ½ cup of chopped onions to the pan, followed by your ¼ cup of chopped garlic. Now stir the ingredients together vigorously as they cook over the course of the next 5 minutes. Scoop the contents into your 3 leaves of lettuce and serve when ready.

Chicken, Vegetables, and Ginger

This lunchtime feast has just the right amount of ginger! It also has just the right amount of onion, just the right amount of garlic, and just the right amount of green bell pepper! It all comes together for this Chicken, Vegetables, and Ginger recipe!

Here are the exact ingredients:

¼ cup of olive oil

¼ cup of chopped garlic

½ cup of chopped onion

¼ cup of powdered ginger

1 cup of chopped chicken breast

½ cup of chicken broth

¼ cup of chopped green bell pepper

¼ cup of celery

Pour your ¼ cup of olive oil into a medium sized frying pan and set your stove's burner for high heat.

Now add your ¼ cup of chopped garlic, your ½ cup of chopped onion, your cup of chopped chicken breast, your ½ cup of chicken broth, your ¼ cup of chopped green bell pepper and your 14 cups of celery/ stir these ingredients together as they cook over the course of the next 5 to 7 minutes. Finally add your ¼ cup of powdered ginger and stir this ingredient into the mix as well. Lunch is served!

Paleo Fish Sticks

Fish sticks are a common staple and a comfort food. They provide an ample amount of protein and other important vitamins and minerals, and this recipe is especially spruced up for the 30-Day Paleo Challenge!

Here are the exact ingredients:

¼ cup of olive oil

5 white fish fillet strips

¼ cup of coconut flour

¼ cup of salt

¼ cup of pepper

½ cup of almond meal

½ cup of ground walnuts

1 eggs

Get out a cooking sheet and evenly coat it with your ¼ cup of olive oil and set it to the side. Now get out a medium sized mixing bowl and add your ¼ cup of coconut flour, your ¼ cup of garlic salt, your ¼ cup of pepper, your ½ cup of almond meal, and your ½ cup of ground walnuts. Take a moment to stir these ingredients together thoroughly. Now get out a small glass bowl or plastic container and crack your 2 eggs into it.

Stir the eggs together well before pouring them into your mixing bowl of other ingredients. Now stir the entire bowl together. Take your fish fillet strips and dip them into your mixture until they are thoroughly coated. Next, place these fish strips onto your olive oil greased cooking pan, place it in the oven and set the temperature to 450 degrees. Cook for about 15 minutes and serve when ready.

Chicken Alfredo Paleo

If you love chicken alfredo, just get a load of Chicken Alfredo Paleo! Instead of filling you up on a bunch of carbs like other pasta, this Chicken Alfredo makes use of kelp noodles, in order to make sure you don't step out of bounds during your 30 Day Paleo Challenge. Keep this recipe on hand for when you need it!

Here are the exact ingredients:

1 cup of chopped chicken breast

1 cup of kelp noodles

½ cup of chopped garlic

½ cup of olive oil

¼ cup of tarragon

1 cup of cashews

¼ cup of onion powder

½ cup of chopped garlic

¼ cup of garlic powder

¼ cup of sea salt

¼ cup of pepper

¼ cup of paprika

Get out a large frying pan and add your ½ cup of olive oil, your ½ cup of chopped garlic, followed by your cup of chopped chicken breast. Now briefly rinse off your cup of kelp noodles and add them to the pan as well. Next, add your ¼ cup of tarragon, and stir the ingredients together well. Put the lid on the pan and let it cook on medium heat for about 15 minutes.

After that you can turn your burner off and drain the oil out of the pan and into a separate container. Save this oil for later, because it can be used as dressing. Next, add your cup of cashews, your ¼ cup of onion powder, your ¼ cup of garlic powder, your ¼ cup of mustard powder, your ¼ cup of sea salt, your ¼ cup of pepper, and your ¼ cup of paprika to a blender.

Put the lid on your blender and blend these ingredients together. Turn the blender off, take off the lid and pour the container of drained oil you saved earlier into the blender. Put the lid back on and blend the ingredients one more time on low speed. Turn blender off again, take off the lid and now pour the contents of the blender into your pan of chicken and other ingredients. Cook on medium heat for about 5 to7 minutes and Paleo lunch is ready to eaten!

Mushroom Leaf Tacos

Need something good to eat for Taco Tuesday? Well look no further my friends! This recipe provides you with a unique and refreshing mix of Paleo ingredients, all coming together to make some of the best tacos you have ever had. So yes, go ahead and try these Mushroom Tacos!

Here are the exact ingredients:

1 cup of chopped mushrooms

1 cup of chopped onions

½ cup of ground beef

¼ cup of red chili pepper

¼ cup of chopped garlic

4 large lettuce leaves

¼ cup of cilantro

Go ahead and set your oven to 400 degrees. While your oven heats up, get out a large frying pan and place your cup of chopped onions inside of it. Set the burner on high. Next, add your cup of chopped mushrooms to the frying pan. Stir these ingredients together as they cook over the next few minutes, before adding your ½ cup of ground beef, your ¼ cup of red chili pepper, and your ¼ cup of chopped garlic.

Cook these ingredients together for about five more minutes. Once cooked, transfer a spoonful of the ingredients onto a spread-out lettuce leaf and then fold the leaf like a taco. The leaves should be sturdy enough to have them filled with ingredients, and then stand them up slightly on their side. Repeat this process with your three other leaves. Your Mushroom Leaf Tacos are ready to eat!

Paleo Meatloaf

Some meatloaf that came straight out of the Paleolithic Era! Our ancestors would have just loved this fine feast! Put this Paleo Meatloaf together and take it to lunch with you! You'll love it!

Here are the exact ingredients:

½ cup of chopped zucchini

¼ cup of chopped carrots

¼ cup peas

½ cup chopped onions

1 pound of mince meat

¼ cup of Italian herbs

¼ cup of salt

1 egg

Set your oven to 350 degrees. Now add your ½ cup of chopped zucchini, your ¼ cup of chopped carrots, your ¼ cup of peas, your ½ cup of chopped onions, and your pound of mincemeat into big mixing bowl and stir all of these ingredients together. Now get out a muffin tray and put a paper muffin cup in each of the tin's six holes.

Now sprinkle your ¼ cup of Italian herbs and your ¼ cup of salt on top of each muffin. Take your (clean) hands and pack your mince meat mixture into each of your paper muffin cups and place your muffin tin into the oven. They should be done after about a half hour, or until the tops of the muffins are brown. Allow the muffin tin to cool off, and eat!

Fried Asparagus and Shiitake Mushrooms

This food tastes as good as it looks! Cooked in oil and apple cider vinegar, this dish has quite a refined taste. Fried Asparagus and Shiitake Mushrooms are your ticket to paleo food paradise!

Here are the exact ingredients:

1 cup of chopped shiitake mushrooms

½ cup of chopped asparagus

¼ cup of olive oil

¼ cup of apple cider vinegar

Coat a frying pan with your ¼ cup of olive oil and set your burner on high. After 2 to 4 minutes you can then add your cup of chopped shitake mushrooms and your ¼ cup of apple cider vinegar. Drain your pan and empty the contents into a plastic container, allow to cool, and serve when ready.

Paleo Roasted Tomatoes

These roasted tomatoes will be the life of the party! Cherry tomatoes cooked in oil, and topped with rosemary and chives. Anyone who sees this dish will be amazed. Even if your family and friends are not themselves a part of the 30-Day Paleo Challenge, they too will love your Paleo Roasted Tomatoes.

Here are the exact ingredients:

Chopped cherry tomatoes

¼ cup of olive oil

¼ cup of chopped rosemary leaves

¼ cup of chopped chives

Get out a medium sized mixing bowl and add your ½ cup of chopped cherry tomatoes, followed by your ¼ cup of olive oil, your ¼ cup of chopped rosemary leaves, and your ¼ cup of chopped chives. Mix together well and then transfer to a frying pan. Set the burner on high, stir, and cook for about 10 minutes. And these Paleo Roasted Tomatoes are ready to go!

Paleo Pork Chops

You can test your finely-honed paleo chops with these Paleo Pork Chops! Cooked with a dash of pepper, salt, and ginger, these chops get the balance right, and will have you licking your own chops in the process! As you can see, paleo can offer up some mighty fine pork chops indeed!

Here are the exact ingredients:

¼ cup of olive oil

¼ cup of salt

¼ cup of pepper

2 lean pork chops

½ cup of water

¼ cup of ginger

¼ cup of crushed, dried rosemary

Place a medium sized frying pan on high heat and coat the bottom of it with your ¼ cup of olive oil. Now get out a small mixing bowl and add your ¼ cup of salt, your ¼ cup of pepper, and your ¼ cup of ginger. Stir these ingredients together well. Now add your ingredients to your pan of oil and place your 2 pork chops into the pan. Add your ½ cup of water and cook the meat for about 2 minutes on each side. Turn off your burner and add your ¼ cup of rosemary on top. Serve when ready.

Pepper Paleo Steaks

Do you love a good steak? Or perhaps a better question is—who doesn't? Well, with a dash of pepper, these paleo steaks have it made in the shade! Bite right into this well cooked meat and taste the result of carefully crafted ingredient put together in perfect harmony.

Here are the exact ingredients:

½ cup of olive oil

¼ cup of garlic powder

¼ cup of paprika

¼ cup of dried thyme

¼ cup of oregano

¼ cup of black pepper

¼ cup of salt

¼ cup of lemon pepper

¼ cup of cayenne pepper

2 beef rib eye steaks

Get out a large mixing bowl and add your ½ cup of olive oil, your ¼ cup of garlic powder, your ¼ cup of paprika, your ¼ cup of dried thyme, your ¼ cup of black pepper, your ¼ cup of salt, your ¼ cup of lemon pepper, your ¼ cup of cayenne pepper, and your ¼ cup of oregano.

Now take out your 2 beef rib eye steaks and put them in a medium sized frying pan and pour the contents of your mixing bowl on top of them. Set your burner on high heat and allow the contents of your pan to cook for about 5 minutes on each side. Turn your oven off. Allow to cool for a few moments and transfer to a plastic container. Put a lid on it and store in your refrigerator.

Paleo Troll Rolls

Despite what the internet trolls may have told you, Paleo Troll Rolls are delicious! And they could be a great part of your lunch routine! Smartly composed of an almond flour mixture, these rolls are completely paleo friendly and taste great.

Here are the exact ingredients:

2 cups of almond flour

¼ cup of baking powder

¼ cup of salt

½ cup of butter

½ cup of water

4 eggs

Set your oven to 400 degrees, and add your ½ cup of butter evenly to each compartment of your muffin tin. Now get out a small mixing bowl and add your 2 cups of almond flour, your ¼ cup of baking powder, and your ¼ cup of salt together, into the bowl. Follow this up by adding your ½ cup of water and your 4 eggs to the mix.

Stir these ingredients together well. Now add the ingredients to your muffin tin and put inside the oven. Allow them to cook for about 15 minutes. During this time the rolls should rise and turn brown. After 15 minutes have passed, take the tin out of the oven, allow the rolls to cool for a moment, and enjoy!

Lamb Kebabs

We live some pretty busy lives and it can be hard to find enough time even to take care of ourselves. But during the lunch time rush, you don't worry to worry have so much about keeping pace, because these Lamb Kebabs will put a smile on your face!

Here are the exact ingredients:

12 rosemary sprigs

1 cup of chopped lamb

¼ cup of honey

¼ cup of olive oil

Place a medium sized frying pan onto a burner set for high heat. Pick your leaves from your rosemary sprigs and place them into your frying pan. Now save your sprigs and put them to the side for later use as your skewers. Next, add your ¼ cup of honey, and your cup of chopped lamb to the pan and allow it to cook for a few minutes. Turn off your burner and put your chunks of chopped lamb onto the skewers. And that's it! Enjoy your Lamb Kebabs!

Moroccan Roast Chicken

This recipe provides some great international flair to your lunchtime needs. You don't have to go to Morocco for this dish, because this paleo friendly chicken is roasted to perfection!

Here are the exact ingredients:

¼ cup of ras el hanout

¼ cup of olive oil

¼ cup of lemon juice

½ cup of chopped chicken

Set your oven to 400 degrees. Now get out a medium sized mixing bowl and add your ¼ cup of ras el hanout, your ¼ cup of olive oil, your ¼ cup of lemon juice, and stir them together well. Now add your ½ cup of chopped chicken to a cooking sheet and marinate it with your mixing bowl of ingredients. Place the pan into the oven and allow it to cook over the next 10 minutes. After your 10 minutes have passed, simply allow to cool, and serve when ready.

Paleo Tuna Stack

If you love tuna, you will love this Paleo Tuna Stack! This delicious blend of tuna is not to be missed! Pack a batch of this recipe in your lunch box!

Here are the exact ingredients:

1 cup of chopped tuna

¼ cup of hot sauce

1 cup of chopped green onions

1 cup of chopped avocado

¼ cup of lemon juice

¼ cup of chopped mango

¼ cup of sesame seeds

¼ cup of coconut aminos

¼ cup of wine vinegar

¼ cup of lemon juice

¼ cup of sesame oil

¼ cup of honey

Let's put together what will amount to your dressing first. Get out a small mixing bowl and add your ¼ cup of sesame seeds, your ¼ cup of coconut aminos, your ¼ cup of lemon juice, your ¼ cup of sesame oil, and your ¼ cup of honey. Mix these ingredients together well and set them to the side for now. Allow these ingredients to settle in for a moment before moving on to the next step.

After you have done this, you can then add your cup of chopped tuna to an additional container and garnish it with your ¼ cup of hot sauce. Now add your cup of chopped green onions, followed by your cup of chopped avocado. Now add your ¼ cup of lemon juice to the bowl and mix it together as well. Finally, take your small bowl of dressing and pour it on top of this bowl of main ingredients. Let this all settle in for a moment and your Paleo Tuna Stack is ready!

Chapter 4: Paleo Dinners on Demand

As the work day draws to a close, for many of us, feeling tired, and hungry we run straight to fridge and end up eating much more than we should. And much of what we eat are things that we shouldn't. We load up on carbs and comfort foods without much of a second's thought about what we are doing to our bodies. But if you stick to the 30-day paleo challenge there are plenty of great and satisfying foods you can eat for your dinner routine. Here are just a few of them!

Lean Beef Stroganoff

This recipe provides you with great protein and great taste. If you like beef that is lean and filling, then Lean Beef Stroganoff certainly fits that billing!

Here are the exact ingredients:

¼ cup of olive oil

½ pound of grass fed beef

½ cup of chopped onion

½ cup of chopped mushrooms

¼ cup of chopped garlic

¼ cup of salt

¼ cup of pepper

1 cup of coconut milk

¼ cup of arrowroot

1 cup of kelp noodles

2 cups of water

Place a large saucepan on a burner set for high heat and add your ¼ cup of olive oil. Now add your ½ cup of chopped onion, and your ½ pound of grass fed beef. Stir these ingredients into the oil as they cook over the next 2 or 3 minutes. You can now add your ½ cup of chopped mushrooms, your ¼ cup of chopped garlic, your ¼ cup of salt, and your ¼ cup of pepper.

Stir in these ingredients as well, and then turn your burner off. Now take out a small pot and add your cup of kelp noodles, your 2 cups of water, and your ¼ cup of arrowroot. Set the burner on high and boil your noodles for about 5 minutes. After this, you can drain the water and dump the noodles into your saucepan and mix it with your other ingredients. Your Lean Beef Stroganoff is complete!

Chicken Paleo Bowl

Chopped red onions, celery, bell pepper, and chicken cooked in coconut oil. This is one big bowl of chicken paleo goodness! Give this recipe a try!

Here are the exact ingredients:

¼ cup of coconut oil

¼ of chopped red onion

¼ cup of chopped celery

¼ cup of chopped green bell peppers

¼ cup of chopped red bell peppers

1 cup of chopped chicken

Put your ¼ cup of coconut oil into a medium sized frying pan and set your burner to high heat. Now add your ¼ cup of chopped red onion, your ¼ cup of chopped celery, your ¼ cup of chopped green bell peppers, your ¼ cup of chopped red bell peppers and your cup of chopped chicken. Stir all of these ingredients together as they cook over the course of the next 5 to 7 minutes and serve when ready.

Asparagus and Beef Stir Fry

Good stir fry can sometimes be hard to come by. And as we are looking for a good dinner at the end of our day, the choices presented to us are not always the best. But this recipe is a game changer, and if you like Stir Fry, then you will love this Paleo Stir Fry treat!

Here are the exact ingredients:

¼ cup of coconut oil

¼ cup of sesame oil

½ pound of grass fed beef

1 cup of chopped onion

1 cup of chopped red bell pepper

½ cup of chopped asparagus

½ cup of chopped garlic

¼ cup of chopped ginger

¼ cup lemon juice

¼ cup of pepper

Get out a large frying, add your ¼ cup of coconut oil and your ¼ cup of sesame oil to the pan. Set your burner on high heat and then add your cup of chopped onion, your cup of chopped red bell pepper, and your ½ cup of chopped asparagus to the pan. Stir these ingredients together as they cook over the next three minutes. Now add your ½ cup of chopped garlic, your ¼ cup of chopped ginger, your ¼ cup of lemon juice, and your ¼ cup of pepper. Put your pan on low heat and allow it to simmer for a few more minutes before turning your burner off and serving.

Chicken and Chile Hash

This dish can hash it out with the best of them! With just the right amount of salt and red pepper, this hearty meal makes for a perfect paleo dinner!

Here are the exact ingredients:

¼ cup of water

¼ cup of olive oil

¼ cup of kosher salt

¼ cup of red pepper

½ cup of ground chicken

½ cup of chopped red onion

½ cup o chopped poblano chilis

1 cup of chopped mushrooms

¼ cup of thyme

½ cup of chopped garlic

¼ cup of red wine vinegar

3 eggs

Place a large frying pan on a burner set to high heat and add ¼ cup of olive oil to the pan, followed by your ¼ cup of kosher salt. Next add your ¼ cup of red pepper, and your ½ cup of ground chicken. Allow these ingredients to cook for about 5 minutes. Follow this up by adding your ½ cup of chopped red onion, your ½ cup of chopped poblano chilis, and your cup of chopped mushrooms in the pan and stir these ingredients together well as they cook over the next 5 to 10 minutes.

Paleo Stir Fry

Here is another great stir fry recipe. If you love eating healthy and you love eating good. Then you just have to check out this stir fry blast from the paleolithic past!

Here are the exact ingredients:

¼ cup of fish sauce

¼ cup of water

¼ cup of lime juice

¼ cup of tomato paste

¼ cup of coconut palm sugar

¼ cup of tabasco sauce

¼ cup of tamari

½ cup of apple cider vinegar

¼ cup of salt

½ cup of white pepper

¼ cup of coconut oil

½ cup of chopped garlic

1 cup of shrimp

½ cup of chopped onion

¼ cup of pineapple

½ cup of chopped tomatoes

½ cup of chopped green bell peppers

Get out a large frying pan and add your ¼ cup of fish sauce, your ¼ cup of water, your ¼ cup of lime juice, your ¼ cup of tomato paste, your ¼ cup of coconut palm sugar, your ¼ cup of tabasco sauce and your ¼ cup of tamri. Now set your burner on low to medium heat, stir well and let simmer. Now get out a medium sized mixing bowl and add your ½ cup of apple cider vinegar, your ¼ cup of salt, your ½ cup of white pepper, and your ¼ cup of coconut oil.

Follow this by depositing your ½ cup of chopped garlic right on top. Stir all of these ingredients together well before adding them to the pan. Now add your ½ cup of chopped onions, your ¼ cup of chopped pineapple, your ½ cup of chopped tomatoes, and ½ cup of chopped green bell peppers. Stir all of the ingredients together over the next 10 minutes and turn your burner off. Allow to cool and then eat!

Spicy Hot Paleo Chicken

Pepper, salt, honey, oregano, paprika, and red chilies come together to make a smash hit! Providing just the right amount of spice for this paleo feast! Have some Spicy Hot Paleo Chicken for dinner!

Here are the exact ingredients:

½ cup of chopped chicken breast

¼ cup of olive oil

¼ cup of chopped red chilies

¼ cup of sweet paprika

¼ cup of chopped oregano

¼ cup of honey

¼ cup of lemon juice

¼ cup of water

¼ cup of salt

¼ cup of pepper

Place a medium sized frying pan on a burner set on high heat and add your ¼ cup of olive oil. Now add your ¼ cup of chopped red chilies, your ¼ cup of chopped oregano, and your ¼ cup of honey. Allow your ingredients to cook over the next few minutes. Now add your ¼ cup of lemon juice, your ¼ cup of water, your ¼ cup of salt, and your ¼ cup of pepper. Stir these ingredients together well over the next few minutes before turning the burner off. Allow to cool, and serve your food.

Oven Roasted Veggie Dinner

Paleo is great for meat eaters but there is still plenty to love for those who like their veggies, and this recipe proves it! Our Paleo ancestors were hunter gatherers and these roasted veggies would have been readily gathered by our paleo forefathers as well!

Here are the exact ingredients:

1 cup of chopped zucchini

1 cup of chopped summer squash

1 cup of chopped red bell pepper

1 cup of chopped yellow bell pepper

½ cup of chopped asparagus

1 cup of chopped red onion

½ cup of chopped garlic

¼ cup of olive oil

¼ cup of salt

¼ cup of pepper

Chop all of your veggies into small pieces and add them to a medium sized mixing bowl and set them to the side. Now get out a large baking sheet and coat it with your ¼ cup of olive oil. Now go back to your mixing bowl and add your ½ cup of chopped garlic, your ¼ cup of salt, and your ¼ cup of pepper.

Stir all of these ingredients together and then add them to your baking sheet. Put the sheet in the oven and set the temperature to 400 degrees and let cook for about half an hour. After your hour has passed, you can then turn your oven off, allow to cool, and serve when you are ready.

Baked Cajun Catfish

If you like yourself some great seafood, then check out this paleo friendly Baked Cajun Catfish. It flawlessly provides you with just what you need for dinner!

Here are the exact ingredients:

1 cup of chopped catfish

¼ cup of flaxseed oil

¼ cup of olive oil

½ cup of chopped garlic

¼ cup of lemon juice

¼ cup of pepper

¼ cup of cayenne pepper

¼ cup of turmeric

Grease an oven safe baking dish with your ¼ cup of flaxseed oil and your ¼ cup of olive oil. Now dump your cup of chopped catfish into the pan. Next, sprinkle your ¼ cup of lemon juice on top, followed by your ¼ cup of pepper, your ¼ cup of cayenne pepper, and your ¼ cup of turmeric. Set your oven to 350 degrees and cook for about a half hour. Allow to cool and your Baked Cajun Catfish is ready to go.

Gazpacho Dinner

If you are looking for a good meal, dinner time is great with a hearty helping of Gazpacho! This meal is tasty and filling!

Here are the exact ingredients:

½ cup of chopped garlic

¼ cup of chopped onion

¼ cup of chopped cucumber

½ cup of chopped tomato

½ cup of tomato juice

¼ cup of white wine vinegar

¼ cup of salt

¼ cup of pepper

Get out your blender and deposit your ½ cup of chopped garlic, your cup of chopped onion, your ¼ cup of chopped cucumber, and your ½ cup of chopped tomato. Put the lid on your blender and blend your ingredients together for a couple of minutes. Next, pour your blended veggies into a mixing bowl and add your ¼ cup of white wine vinegar, your ¼ cup of salt, and your ¼ cup of pepper on top of the mix. Stir these ingredients together well and then put a lid on the bowl. Put this sealed container into your fridge and let it marinate for at least a half hour before serving.

Spicy Paleo Flounder

Attention fish lovers! This recipe sets out to prove just how good the Paleo Diet really is! Delicious fish and veggies have never been better! Just check out this Spicy Paleo Flounder!

Here are the exact ingredients:

2 cups of chopped flounder

1 cup of chopped garlic

¼ cup of olive oil

¼ cup of dill

¼ cup of turmeric

½ cup of chopped carrots

¼ cup of lemon juice

¼ cup of black pepper

To get started, get out an oven safe baking dish and evenly coat the bottom of it with your ¼ cup of olive oil. Now add your 2 cups of chopped flounder to the dish and sprinkle your ¼ cup of dill, and your ¼ cup of turmeric on top. Next, begin spreading your ½ cup of carrots over the fish.

Then sprinkle your ¼ cup of lemon juice and ¼ cup of black pepper on top. Cover this dish and place in the oven. Set your oven's temperature to 400 degrees and cook for about 20 minutes. After it has cooked, allow it to cool off at room temperature for a few minutes before serving.

Spicy Nigerian Beef

This spicy paleo dinner has a bit of international flair and won't leave you disappointed! Hearty beef sirloin marinated to perfection with just the right kick of jalapeno and habanero peppers! This recipe will be an instant success!

Here are the exact ingredients:

2 cups of beef sirloin

¼ cup of olive oil

¼ cup of onion powder

¼ cup of black pepper

¼ cup of garlic powder

¼ cup of powdered ginger

¼ cup of paprika

¼ cup of chili powder

¼ cup of cayenne pepper

1 cube of chicken bouillon

¼ cup of roasted cashews

¼ cup of chopped tomatoes

¼ cup of chopped onions

¼ cup of chopped jalapeno

¼ cup of chopped habanero

¼ cup of lime juice

½ cup of water

Get out a large mixing bowl and add your 2 cups of chopped beef sirloin, followed by your ¼ cup of garlic powder, your ¼ cup of ginger, and your ¼ cup of paprika. Now get out your blender and add to it your ¼ cup of chili powder, your ¼ cup of cayenne pepper, your ¼ cup of chopped jalapeno, and your ¼ cup of chopped habanero. Pulse these ingredients together, turn it off, and pour them into the mixing bowl of ingredients.

Set these to the side for a moment Put a large frying pan on medium heat and add your ½ cup of water, and your ¼ cup of lime juice. Follow this up by adding your cube of chicken bouillon and stir these ingredients together. Now add your ¼ cup of roasted cashews, your ¼ cup of chopped onions, and your ¼ cup of chopped tomatoes, stir these ingredients together as they cook over the next few minutes.

Now go back to the spicy beef mixture in your mixing bowl and add it to your pan as well. Stir everything together as it cooks over the next 5 minutes. Now turn your burner off and allow it all to cool. You are now ready to serve up some seriously spicy, and seriously delicious, Spicy Nigerian Beef!

Paleo Pan Fried Garlic Calamari

Paleo Pan Fried Garlic Calamari is a uniquely delicious dish! Chopped squid cooked in olive oil and garnished with a hearty helping of garlic. Don't underestimate the power of this recipe!

Here are the exact ingredients:

1 cup of chopped calamari squid

½ cup of olive oil

½ cup of chopped garlic

½ cup of chopped parsley

Add your cup of chopped calamari along with your ½ cup of olive oil and your ½ cup of chopped garlic. Stir together well and then transfer to a frying pan. Set your burner on high, and stir fry your ingredients for a few minutes before adding your ½ cup of chopped parsley and turn your burner off. Serve when ready.

Thyme-Braised Short Ribs Dinner

These short ribs are incredible! This dish is braised to perfection!

Here are the exact ingredients:

¼ cup of coconut oil

2 pounds beef short ribs

¼ cup of salt

¼ cup of pepper

1 cup of chopped onion

¼ cup of chopped carrots

½ cup of chopped celery

½ cup of chopped garlic

¼ cup of tomato paste

¼ cup of balsamic vinegar

½ cup of water

3 cups of beef broth

7 Portobello mushroom caps

Start off by sprinkling your ribs with your ¼ cup of salt, and your ¼ cup of pepper. Now place a pot on a burner and set it to high heat. Add your ¼ cup of coconut oil to the pot. Place your ribs into the pot on top of this layer of coconut oil. Next add your cup of chopped onion, your ¼ cup of chopped carrots, your ½ cup of chopped celery, as well as your ½ cup of chopped garlic to the pot.

Stir the ingredients together and allow them to cook for about 5 minutes. After this add your ½ cup of tomato paste, your ¼ cup of balsamic vinegar, your ½ cup of water, and your 3 cups of beef broth to the pot. Stir, and let these ingredients boil for another 5 minutes. After this time has passed, turn your burner off, drain the pot of liquid and dump your ingredients into a large baking pan.

Spread all of these ingredients out evenly and then layer your 7 Portobello mushroom caps on top of the ingredients. Now place your pan of ingredients into the oven and set the temperature to 400 degrees.

Allow the ingredients to roast in the oven for about 10 minutes and then turn the oven off. Scoop the contents onto a large plate and your dinner is ready!

The Wild Duck Burger

Wild game was a common source of nutrition for our Paleolithic ancestors. Any wild birds of the field they could find would have served as a lovely dinner for them. In this recipe we take that bird meat and make it into a burger that most of us would enjoy today. This Wild Duck Burger tastes really fantastic. Just slap some lettuce buns on that bad boy and dinner is ready!

Here are the exact ingredients:

1 cup of chopped duck

½ cup of chopped garlic

½ cup of chopped onions

¼ cup of chopped tomatoes

4 to 6 crisp pieces of lettuce

¼ cup of salt

1 egg

Dump your cup of chopped duck into a meat grinder and grind it down to a fine paste. Once it's all ground up, deposit your meat into a large mixing bowl. Now add your egg, your ½ cup of chopped garlic, your ½ cup of chopped onions, your ¼ cup of chopped tomatoes, and your ¼ cup of salt to the mixing bowl and stir it all up together.

Once stirred, begin shaping the mixture into patty-form. You should be able to make at least 3 or 4 solid duck patties with them. Place these into a large frying pan, set the burner on high and cook each side for about 5 minutes or until brown. Allow your duck burgers to cool and then deposit them between a couple leaves of crisp lettuce. Serve when you are ready.

Beef Cabbage Rolls

If you like your beef, then you are going to love Paleo. The Paleo diet is full of all kinds of beef based meals to choose from. This next recipe is no exception to this rule. Check out this tasty lean beef garnished with garlic, onions and tomatoes, these Beef Cabbage Rolls are going to be a smash hit!

Here are the exact ingredients:

1 head of cabbage

1 pound of lean ground beef

1 cup of chopped onions

¼ cup of black pepper

¼ cup of chopped garlic

½ cup of chopped tomatoes

¼ cup of oregano

2 eggs

For starters, take your cabbage and remove its core. Now steam the whole head of cabbage for a few minutes until the leaves loosen up and fall right off. Take these leaves and put them on a large plate for the moment and keep them to the side. Now get out a medium sized mixing bowl and add your pound of lean ground beef, and your cup of chopped onions.

Follow this up by adding your ¼ cup of black pepper, your ¼ cup of chopped garlic, your ½ cup of chopped tomatoes, your ¼ cup of oregano, and your 2 eggs to the bowl. After you have added all of these ingredients together mix them well and transfer them to a frying pan. Set the pan on high heat and cook the ingredients for about 10 minutes while you stir them together. Turn off the burner.

Now take your leaves and spread them out on a large baking dish. Transfer a spoonful of your cooked meat ingredients to each opened leave in the baking dish. Fold the leaves over inside the dish, and place them in the oven. Set your oven to 400 degrees. Allow these

Beef Cabbage Rolls to cook for about an hour and serve when ready.

Chapter 5: A Few Special Side Dishes and other Paleo Recipes

Paleo has just as many great side dishes as it does main course meals. There are a countless variety of soups, salads, snacks, and sides that you can enjoy during your 30-day paleo challenge. Each one has its own unique purpose and strengths. Her are a few of the best.

Chicken Avocado Soup

With juicy bits of chicken cooked to perfection along with all your favorite veggies, Chicken Avocado Soup is always a good recipe to have on hand.

Here are the exact ingredients:

2 cups of chopped chicken

1 cup of chicken broth

½ cup of chopped onion

¼ cup of chopped celery

¼ cup of rosemary

½ cup of chopped avocado

¼ cup of chopped cilantro

To get started, toss your cup of chopped chicken, your 2 cups of chicken broth, your ½ cup of chopped onion, your ¼ cup of chopped celery, and your ¼ cup of chopped cilantro into a medium sized saucepan and set your burner to high heat. Stir these ingredients as they cook over the next few minutes. Next, sprinkle your ¼ cup of rosemary, your ½ cup of chopped avocado, and your ¼ cup of chopped cilantro on top. Stir all of these ingredients together one final time before turning your burner off. Your Chicken Avocado soup is ready to eat.

Paleo Kale Chips

We all love to snack on potato chips from time to time, but these heavily processed foods are not good for our bottom line. Fortunately for us however, Paleo offers us a great alternative in the form of Paleo Kale Chips. These chips are salty and fulfilling, without all the baggage that comes with junk food. So, if you have a craving for a good snack, just give this recipe a try!

Here are the exact ingredients:

1 cup of chopped kale

½ cup of olive oil

¼ cup of sea salt

Set your oven to about 350 degrees. Now take your chopped kale and make sure that all of the stems are removed. You want your chopped pieces to primarily consist of the leaves of the Kale plant. Now add your cup of chopped kale to a medium sized mixing bowl followed by your ½ cup of olive oil. Stir these ingredients together well before laying all of your kale out on a cooking sheet and putting them into your oven. Allow these kale chips to cook for about 10 minutes or until they are nice and crispy! Now you are ready for your next snack attack!

Paleo Cream Soup

Tasty asparagus, soaked in coconut butter and chicken broth. This is soothing paleo comfort food at its best, and this Paleo Cream Soup more than passes the paleolithic test!

Here are the exact ingredients:

1 cup of chopped asparagus

1 cup of chicken broth

¼ cup of salt

¼ cup of pepper

¼ cup of coconut butter

¼ cup of coconut milk

First, fill up a microwave safe container with your cup of chicken broth. After you have done this you can then cover the dish with some plastic wrap and cook your broth in the microwave for about 2 minutes. After warming it up like this, transfer the contents of the dish to a blender and place to the side for the moment. Now put your cup of chopped asparagus into the microwave safe container along with your cup of chicken broth and warm it up for 2 to 3 minutes.

Take out your container of broth and asparagus and dump it into your blender. Now add your ¼ cup of coconut butter, and your ¼ cup of coconut milk and blend everything together. Turn off the blender and pour the blended ingredients into a medium sized saucepan. Place the pan on low heat and allow to simmer for about a half hour before serving.

Artichoke Heart Salad

You can eat your heart on this salad because this is a hefty recipe that works well for any day of your 30-day challenge!

Here are the exact ingredients:

1 cup of chopped artichoke hearts

1 cup of chopped red bell pepper

1 cup of chopped onion

½ cup of lemon juice

¼ cup of olive oil

¼ cup of pepper

¼ cup of salt

½ cup of chopped avocado

First, take your cup of chopped artichoke hearts, your cup of chopped onion, your cup of chopped red bell pepper, your ½ cup of lemon juice, and your ¼ cup of olive oil and mix it all together thoroughly in a small bowl. Now sprinkle your ¼ cup of pepper, and your ¼ cup of salt on top of the mixture. Finally add your ½ cup of chopped avocado on top, and your Artichoke Heart Salad is ready to go. This is one of the best paleo recipes you could possibly come by.

Cucumber Salad

Crunchy cucumbers and tasty blueberries come together to make a real treat. This salad is healthy, satisfying, and a great part of the paleo diet.

Here are the exact ingredients:

2 cucumbers

½ cup of chopped blueberries

½ cup of olive oil

¼ cup of vinegar

¼ cup of feta cheese

To get started on this paleo recipe you need to take your cucumbers, completely peel them and slice them in half lengthwise. And then cut these slices in half one more time. Add these slices to a large mixing bowl and add your ½ cup of chopped blueberries, your ½ cup of olive oil, your ¼ cup of vinegar, and your ¼ cup of feta cheese. Stir these ingredients together well and serve.

Ginger and Carrot Soup

Chopped carrots garnished with garlic, onions, and ground ginger come together perfectly in this recipe. This tasty soup is one of a kind!

Here are the exact ingredients:

4 cups of chopped carrots

¼ cup of olive oil

¼ cup of ground ginger

½ cup of chopped onions

½ cup of chopped garlic

¼ cup of ground turmeric

¼ cup of ground ginger

¼ cup of vegetable stock

¼ cup of coconut milk

Set your oven for 400 degrees. Take out a cooking sheet and coat it with your ¼ cup of olive oil, before adding your ¼ cup of ginger evenly over the cooking sheet. Now add your 4 cups of chopped carrots on the cooking sheet and place in the oven. Allow these ingredients to cook for about a half hour.

While the cooking sheet of ingredients are cooking, place a medium sized frying pan on a burner set for high heat and add your ½ cup of chopped onions, your ½ cup of chopped garlic, your ¼ cup of ground turmeric, your ¼ cup of ground ginger, your ¼ cup of vegetable stock, and your ¼ cup of coconut milk.

Stir these ingredients together well as they cook over the next 5 to 7 minutes. Finally, turn your burner and your oven off and add your cooking sheet ingredients to your pan of ingredients and mix them all together well. This paleo dish is now ready to rock and roll!

Spinach Salad

This Spinach Salad comes complete with chopped strawberries, garlic, vinegar, and olive oil. This is a great salad for the paleo diet; or any other diet for that matter!

Here are the exact ingredients:

1 cup of chopped strawberries

½ cup of olive oil

½ cup of vinegar

½ cup of chopped garlic

½ cup of poppy seeds

¼ cup of black pepper

Add your cup of chopped strawberries, your ½ cup of olive oil, your ½ cup of vinegar, your ½ cup of chopped garlic, your ½ cup of poppy seeds, and your ¼ cup of black pepper to a medium sized mixing bowl. Thoroughly mix these ingredients together and your Spinach Salad is ready to go!

Broccoli Soup

This Broccoli Soup is a great staple to have on hand any time of the day.

Here are the exact ingredients:

½ cup of olive oil

¼ cup of arrowroot

7 cups of vegetable stock

3 cups of chopped broccoli

To prepare this paleo dish, get out a large saucepan and add your ½ cup of olive oil, and your ¼ cup of arrowroot to the bottom of the pan. Now set your burner on high and add your 7 cups of vegetable stock. Stir these ingredients together well before adding your 3 cups of chopped broccoli. Stir these ingredients as they cook over the next half hour. After that, soup's on!

Paleo Cucumber Salad

Another great salad for your 30-Day Paleo Challenge! Cucumber, tomatoes, chopped dill and cider vinegar come together like never before!

Here are the exact ingredients:

1 cup of chopped cucumber

1 cup of chopped tomatoes

¼ cup of apple cider vinegar

¼ cup of chopped dill

For this recipe, its easy. All you really have to do is add all of your ingredients together in a large mixing bowl and stir well. Once you have done this, you just need to cool the ingredients down a bit by leaving them in your fridge to chill for a couple of hours. This will ensure that the veggies are all nice and crisp when you serve them. So just mix it all together in a bowl, put it in your refrigerator to chill, and this paleolithic recipe is complete!

Paleo Cookies

Even during the 30-Day Paleo Challenge you could use a treat, and these Paleo Cookies are the best way to do it! Just mix, bake and serve up this batch of Paleo Cookie goodness!

Here are the exact ingredients:

1 cup of chopped bananas

½ cup of chopped apples

¼ cup of raw chopped walnuts

¼ cup of coconut milk

¼ cup of flax

¼ cup of cinnamon

¼ cup of baking soda

¼ cup of olive oil

Set your oven to 350 degrees. Now take out a medium sized mixing bowl and add your cup of chopped bananas, your ½ cup of chopped apples, and your ¼ cup of chopped walnuts. Stir these ingredients together well before adding your ¼ cup of coconut milk, your ¼ cup of flax, your ¼ cup of cinnamon, and your ¼ cup of baking soda. Stir all of these ingredients together well.

Now get out a cooking sheet and evenly coat it with your ¼ cup of olive oil. Now take your (clean) hands and use them to shape your cookies out of your dough in the mixing bowl. Place these drops of dough onto the cookie sheet. Make sure that they are evenly spaced apart and then place your cooking sheet into the oven. Let the cookies cook for about 15 minutes. These Paleo Cookies are done!

Sweet Paleo Potato Fries

If you really need a pick-me-up, these Sweet Paleo Potato Fries will really hit the spot! Treat yourself with some Sweet Paleo Potato Fries today!

Here are the exact ingredients:

1 cup of chopped sweet potato

1 egg white

¼ cup of chili powder

¼ cup of garlic powder

¼ cup of onion powder

¼ cup of sat

Get out your sweet potatoes and peel them, before chopping them up and depositing them into a mixing bowl. Now add your egg white and stir these ingredients together. Add these ingredients to a medium sized saucepan and add your ¼ cup of chili powder, your ¼ cup of garlic powder, your ¼ cup of onion powder, and your ¼ cup of salt. Turn your burner off and serve when ready.

Paleo Mayonnaise

Paleo Mayonnaise is a super food condiment! This wholesome blend of egg, dry mustard, lemon juice, and olive oil can be used on just about anything! Try this fantastic recipe to stock up on your own!

Here are the exact ingredients:

1 egg

¼ cup of olive oil

¼ cup of lemon juice

¼ cup of cayenne pepper

¼ cup of dry mustard

Put your egg, your ¼ cup of dry mustard, and ¼ cup of olive oil into a blender. Set the blender to puree for a couple of minutes, before stopping the blender and adding ¼ cup of lemon juice. Now close the lid of the blender and hit puree again to blend the contents of the blender once again. Pour the content of the blender into a mixing bowl and add your ¼ cup of cayenne pepper. Stir everything together one more time. The texture of your mayonnaise should now be nice and thick. Just pour it into a glass jar for storage and your Paleo Mayonnaise is complete.

Apple Cherry Crumble Cake

This paleo dessert is a good treat at the end of the day!
Save this recipe for when you really need it!

Here are the exact ingredients:

1 cup of chopped cherries

1 cup of chopped apples

¼ cup of lemon juice

¼ cup of cashews

¼ cup of cinnamon

¼ cup of coconut oil

Set your oven to 350 degrees. Now take your cup of chopped cherries, your cup of chopped apples and put them in an oven safe dish. Now get out a small mixing bowl and add your ¼ cup of lemon juice, your ¼ cup of cashews, your ¼ cup of cinnamon, and your ¼ cup of coconut oil. Mix these ingredients together well and then pour them over your apples and cherries in the dish. Place your dish in the oven and allow it to cook for about a half hour. Once your half hour has passed, turn off your oven and allow the Apple Cherry Crumble Cake to cool.

Butternut Squash Paleo Pear Puree

Ok, so maybe our Paleolithic ancestors didn't have a blender they could set to "Puree" but they did like their butternut squash! And you will too! Check out this amazing recipe!

Here are the exact ingredients:

1 cup of chopped butternut squash

1 cup of chopped pears

¼ cup of salt.

Set your oven to 400 degrees. Now get out a baking dish and place some aluminum foil at the bottom of it. Now add your cup of chopped butternut squash and your cup of chopped pears to the dish, spreading each of these ingredients out evenly. After you have done this, place them in the oven and allow them to cook for about half an hour or until brown.

Once your half hour has passed you can then turn your oven off and dump the ingredients into a blender. Add your ¼ cup of salt to the top of the mixture before putting the lid on the blender and hitting the puree button. Thoroughly blend the up ingredients over the next few minutes. And serve up a side of Butternut Squash Paleo Pear Puree!

Paleolithic Lemon Soufflé

This recipe allows you to make a side dish with some real class! Paleolithic Lemon Soufflé is a great reward for your 30-Day Paleo Challenge!

Here are the exact ingredients:

½ cup of lemon juice

1 scooped out lemon rind

1 cup of coconut milk

¼ cup of honey

3 eggs

Set your oven for 350 degrees. Now get out a medium sized mixing bowl and add your ¼ cup of lemon juice, your ¼ cup of honey, your 3 eggs, and your coconut milk. Mix these together until they constitute one fine paste. Now take your scooped-out lemon rind and put it in the center of a slightly greased cooking sheet. Pour your ingredients into the lemon rind. Now put the cooking sheet in the oven and allow it to cook for about 15 minutes until the soufflé rises. Your Paleolithic Lemon Soufflé is now ready for business.

Paleo Pocket Popsicles

With its great taste and its close adherence to the guidelines of the 30-Day Paleo Challenge, this recipe is a true delight! Paleo Pocket Popsicles are easy to make and even easier to eat!

Her are the exact ingredients:

4 cups of coconut water

½ cup of lime juice

¼ cup of lime zest

1 cup of chopped raspberries

1 cup of chopped peaches

1 cup of coconut milk

½ cup of lemon juice

1 cup of chopped blueberries

Take 12 Dixie cups and put them on a cooking sheet. Now mix your ingredients together in a mixing bowl and deposit the mixture into each of the Dixie cups.

Now stick a straw in the center of each one of the mixtures. Place in the freezer and allow to freeze over the next few hours. You can now go ahead and pocket these popsicles!

Banana Pudding

With recipes like this the 30-Day Paleo Challenge isn't a challenge at all! This banana pudding is hands down the best paleo friendly pudding in town!

Here are the exact ingredients:

1 cup of chopped banana

¼ cup of coconut milk

¼ cup of chia seeds

¼ cup of vanilla extract

Add your cup of chopped banana and your ¼ cup of coconut milk to a blender, shut the lid, and thoroughly blend together. Next, take the lid off and add your ¼ cup of chia seeds to the mix. Shut the lid again, and pulse the blender a few more times just to mix the seeds into the rest of the ingredients.

Now transfer the contents of your blender to a mixing bowl and add your ¼ cup of vanilla extract. Stir all of these ingredients together well. Put a lid on the mixing bowl and place it in the fridge to settle. After about an hour or so, take out of the fridge and serve.

Chapter 6: Refreshing Recipes for Paleo Beverages

One of the biggest complaints that many have when it comes to starting the Paleo Challenge is quite often not over the food they have to eat, but over the drinks that they have to give up. Many are disappointed when they have to put their favorite sodas, Frappuccino's, and energy drinks to the side. For many it is losing these beverages that constitutes the greatest sacrifice of all.

But you just because you have to get rid of some of these overly processed beverages, doesn't mean you can't have some suitable alternatives. And just in case you are someone who tends to be on the thirsty side, you are in like. Because we have a plethora of great drinks you can enjoy while engaging in, and successfully adhering to, the 30-day paleo challenge.

Ginger Basil Tea

½ cup of ground coriander

¼ cup of ground cardamom

¼ cup of black pepper

¼ cup of grated ginger

½ cup of honey

4 cups of water

1 lime sliced

8 fresh basil leaves

Take out a small sauce pan and add your ½ cup of ground coriander, and your ¼ cup of ground cardamom, followed by your black pepper. Now set your burner to low heat and stir and cook these ingredients for about 4 minutes. Next, get out a medium sized saucepan and add your ½ cup of honey, your 4 cups of water, your ¼ cup of grated ginger, your 1 slice of lime, and your 8 fresh basil leaves.

Set your burner for medium heat, stir and let all of these ingredients cook over the next 10 minutes. Allow to cool for a minute or two before draining your tea into a pitcher. Let your tea stand at room temperature, or chill it in the fridge for about a half hour before serving. Your Ginger Basil Tea is now ready to drink!

Paleo Apple Tea

With just two apples, some cinnamon, and three teabags, this Paleo Apple Tea really hits the spot!

Here are the exact ingredients:

2 medium apples

3 teabags

¼ cup of cinnamon

Completely peel your apples and then cut them up into small pieces. Now pour your 5 cups of water down into a cooking pot and set the burner on high. You can now add your cup of chopped apples, and your ¼ cup of cinnamon to the pot. Stir these together well before taking your burner down to low heat and allowing the contents of the pan to simmer.

Put a lid on the pot and let it simmer like this over the course of the next couple of hours. Now pour the liquid into a large (and cleaned out) milk jug and store in your fridge over the next few hours. While in the refrigerator the ingredients will settle and congeal together. After this your Paleo Apple Tea is ready to drink!

Paleo Energy Drink

If you love your caffeine like I do, then you probably are known to reach for those store-bought energy drinks from time to time. The only trouble is; those standard energy drinks can wreak havoc on your paleo diet. Check out this recipe for a safe alternative that tastes good, keeps you awake, and won't mess up your 30-day paleo challenge! Just take it from me, if you feel yourself slumping over and falling asleep at the tail end of a long workday or work project, this Paleo Drink will send you into high gear!

Here are the exact ingredients:

1 cup of coconut water

1 cup of chopped watermelon

½ cup of lime

¼ cup of sea salt

This one is about as straightforward as it gets. Simply add your cup of coconut water, your cup of chopped watermelon, your ½ cup of lime, and your ¼ cup of sea salt to a blender, put a lid on, and blend all of the ingredients together well. Now just pour it in a glass and serve up some of that great Paleo energy!

Cucumber Lime Water

Cucumber Lime Water is one of my favorite paleo drinks. When cucumber and lime come together like it does in this recipe, it makes for quite a refreshing taste!

Here are the exact ingredients:

1 cucumber

1 lime

2 cups of water

Start off by peeling the skin off your cucumbers and then chopping it into really thin pieces. Next, add your pieces to an empty (and thoroughly cleaned out) milk or water jug. Add your ½ cup of lime to the jug, followed by your 3 cups of water. Put the lid on your jug and shake it all up as hard as you can. After shaking up these ingredients thoroughly, put the jug of ingredients inside of your refrigerator and let it settle in place over the next 24 hours. The next day your refreshing cucumber lime water is ready to drink!

Paleo Coconut Water Smoothie

You can make a really great smoothie just out of coconut water. And this recipe serves as a fantastic staple of the paleo diet. Try yourself a Paleo Coconut Water Smoothie today!

Here are the exact ingredients:

1 cup of coconut water

1 banana

¼ cup of cashews

½ cup of spinach

¼ cup of coconut oil

¼ cup of potato starch

Get out your blender and add your cup of coconut water inside. Follow this by adding your banana, your coconut oil, your ½ cup of spinach, your ¼ cup of cashews, and your ¼ cup of potato starch. Close the lid on your blender and hit the button to turn it on. Blend everything together well.

Almond Butter Chocolate Shake

Smoother than a smoothie, this shake goes down well at the end of any Paleo day! This Almond Butter Chocolate Shake is good I every way!

1 cup of chopped banana

½ cup of homemade milk

½ cup of almond butter

¼ cup of vanilla extract

¼ cup of cacao powder

¼ cup of salt

4 ice cubes

Place your cup of chopped bananas, your ½ cup of homemade milk, your ½ cup of almond butter, your ¼ cup of vanilla extract, your ¼ cup of cacao powder, and your ¼ cup of salt into a blender. Add your 4 ice cubes on top of these ingredients, close the lid and blend. After a few minutes you should have a very refreshing Almond Butter Chocolate Shake indeed.

Paleo Pumpkin Coffee

Now that fall is here, everyone wants Pumpkin Coffee. You see folks lining up in coffee joints such as Starbucks eager to get their hands on their hands on pumpkin spice lattes and the like. But you don't have to line up to get a good pumpkin flavored coffee, and you don't have to fork over 5 dollars a cup for that matter either. Because you can make your own Paleo Pumpkin Coffee right out of your own home. So here it is folks, for your pumpkin flavored coffee consumption; Paleo Pumpkin Coffee!

Here are the exact ingredients:

1 cup of black coffee

¼ cup of pumpkin puree

¼ cup of cinnamon

¼ cup of nutmeg

¼ cup of cloves

¼ cup of ghee

Take your cup of black coffee and pour it into a standard blender. Now take your ¼ cup of pumpkin puree, your ¼ cup of cinnamon, your ¼ cup of nutmeg, your ¼ cup of cloves, and your ¼ cup of ghee and add these to the blender as well. Now simply press the button to blend, and once blended, pour contents into a coffee cup. Finally, put this cup of mixed coffee ingredients into the microwave and allow it to heat up for about 45 seconds. Your Paleo Pumpkin Cofree is ready.

Coconut Ice Cream Shake

This smooth blend of coconut milk goes down about as easy as it is to make it! Try this recipe today!

Here are the exact ingredients:

1 cup of coconut milk

1 cup of chopped fruit

¼ cup of vanilla

All you have to do is add your coconut milk to your blender, followed by your cup of chopped fruit and your ¼ cup vanilla, and then turn the blender on. Let the ingredients blend for just a minute or so and then turn your blender off and transfer the blended contents to a small container. Put a lid on the container and put it in your refrigerator to chill. After about an hour this Coconut Ice Cream Shake is ready to drink!

Chapter 7: Final Thoughts and Tips to Help You Meet your Challenge!

Besides eating the recipes recommended in this book, there are a few more tips and tricks that could be of service for you, and help you meet your goals even better. Here in this chapter we present to you some final thoughts on how you can meet your 30-day challenge successfully.

Get Enough Exercise

No matter what your diet is, the power of exercise cannot be underestimated. And if you think about it, our Paleolithic Ancestors were a pretty active bunch. They walked several miles a day, were able to outrun wooly mammoths, swam lakes, rivers, and streams looking for fish and climbed trees to get fruit, so we know that they got their exercise! So, having that said, exercise is part and parcel to the paleo challenge.

And although you don't have to outrun a wooly mammoth, you should be able to do some sort of cardio vascular exercise—whether it is going for a walk or just running in place in your own home. All of these exercises are enough to get your heart pumping, and improve your circulation. You should also invest in some upper body strength training such as push-ups, pull ups, or weight lifting. If you get enough exercise your 30-day paleo challenge will be a breeze!

Take the Challenge with a Friend

Everything is just a little bit easier when we have a partner to experience challenges with. And the same goes for the Paleo challenge. If you have a friend or significant other who is interested in changing their diet, you should encourage them to partake in the 30-day paleo challenge right along with you.

That way you can have a constant source of encouragement, even as you help each other along. Besides—that's how our Paleolithic ancestors lived out their lives in the first place. They lived and worked as a team in their efforts to hunt and gather and you can your own personal friend and ally can also work together to successfully complete your 30-day paleo challenge.

Allow Yourself to be Hungry

Hunger is normal. And experiencing hunger in between meals is just part of the metabolic process of your body as it uses up its nutrient resources during the course of a day. Your hunger is just a side effect of this process that alerts you to what your body needs to have replenished. Allow yourself to be hungry so you can witness this mechanism at work.

Get Fresh Air and Sunshine

Our paleo ancestors spent almost all of their time outside. This is where they got their bread and butter through hunting, foraging, and gathering. But today for most of us the reverse is true, for most of us, we spend the majority of our time inside. But we are not so far removed from our paleolithic past that we can't still benefit a great deal from getting a little bit of fresh air and sunshine.

Sunshine itself has been proven beneficial to the human body in the form of the Vitamin D that it bombards us with. Vitamin D helps the body in a wide variety of ways; including the development of bones. So, 30-day paleo challenge or not, in the long run, simply getting some fresh air and sunshine can help you out tremendously.

Get some Sleep

Sleep is an important component of how our body's function and most especially how they metabolize and process the foods that we eat. If you are not getting enough sleep your body will not be able to efficiently take in all of the nutrients you are feeding it. In order to get your body running and humming like a well-oiled machine you are going to have to get some sleep!

Track Your Progress

As you continue on the Paleo diet you need to be as patient as possible as you monitor your progress. Keep track of the small things, and take note of milestones along the way. The Paleo Challenge is more of a marathon than it is a sprint. So be patient and take stock of what you have already accomplished. The more of your success that you see, the more it will encourage you to go forward.

Weight loss is the most obvious form of accomplishment of any diet, but perhaps you can monitor improvements in other areas of your life as well. Do you have less stress towards the end of your 30-day challenge? Do you feel happier? Are those around you beginning to notice a positive shift in direction in your general attitude? These are all potential benefits of the 30-day challenge and well worth nothing as you track your progress.

Experiment with Organs

No, this section is not advising you to become a doctor and experiment with organ transplants! Because when we say "experiment with organs" as it pertains to Paleo means experimenting with organ eats from animals. Although most of us nowadays strictly eat the muscle tissues of livestock, our ancestors got a large part of their nutrition through the consumption of organs such as the hearts, livers, and even lungs, of the animals that they hunted.

Even if you initially turn your nose at the thought, just consider the fact that organ meat from a cow doesn't taste that much different from other meat consumed from the cow's body. Beef hearts taste fairly similar to other kinds of beef, so don't be afraid to experiment. Organs are no doubt the healthiest part of an animal to consume. They are loaded with vitamins and minerals that you can't get any other way. Our paleolithic ancestors loved to eat them, and you should too!

Eat Your Leftover Food

Leftovers get a bad rap but the truth is, they can save you a whole lot of time, energy, and stress! If you have any extra food from lunch that you don't feel like eating, because you are full or pressed for time, don't throw it away. Instead put it in a plastic container and save it for later, that way you can have some fully prepped food ready for you by the time the next day comes around again!

Have a Hobby

We all have hobbies that we gain fulfillment from, but eating should not be one of them! If your hobby is staring at the TV and munching on a big old bag of potato chips we need to correct that part of your routine! You should have plenty of fulfilling hobbies that have nothing at all to do with food in which you can invest your time. That way you will be more likely to eat only when you need nourishment and not just for something to do.

For our Paleolithic ancestors after all, there was no such thing as eating out of boredom, they only ate to survive. For paleo man his downtime was filled with non-food eating activity such as singing, storytelling, cave painting and the like. So, let's go back to those paleo days of yore and find ways to fulfill ourselves without constantly filling our bellies. Find a good hobby.

Become a Good Cook

As this book demonstrates, eating the right foods is only one aspect of a successfully 30-day paleo challenge, since most of the recipes presented in this book requires some basic preparation, you need to be a good cook as well. If you have never cooked much in your life, this book is a great first step for you since the recipes presented here are all fairly straightforward, "no frills" and right to the point. Use this book as a stepping stone in your culinary career and you will indeed become a good cook by the time your 30-day paleo challenge comes to a close.

Drink A Lot of H2O

Considering the fact that our bodies are made up of 98% water, it is really no wonder that we need to have replenishments of this resource on a daily basis. In fact, without new additions of water at least every 3 days, our bodies are unable to continue carrying out their functions. Digestion grinds to a halt without adequate H2O to facilitate the process and our very hearts can't beat as they become water depleted. As you can see, this chemical combination called H2O is very important, so make sure that you drink a lot of it!

Get a Handle on Your Caffeine Intake

As much as we love the smell of that coffee in the morning or perhaps the sudden rush of an energy drink in the evening. We need to get a handle on our caffeine intake. While caffeine in itself is not necessarily harmful to your results on the Paleo Challenge. If you can't even get through the day without downing three energy drinks this is a problem that needs to be created and by forcing your body to reboot and reprogram itself by going 30 days without constantly consuming caffeine, you could greatly benefit in the process.

Quit Smoking

By most accounts our Paleolithic Ancestors did not puff on cigars, cigarettes or hookahs, so in order to properly simulate the conditions of their Paleolithic past you shouldn't either. Smoking will only slow you down. There are so many toxic ingredients in cigarette smoke it will make your head spin. Many smoke because they think that it will help them lose weight.

They see the act of cigarette smoking as an action of negating their cravings for food. But quitting smoking right as you start the paleo challenge is a great tactic because it allows you to end one habit and replace it with another. So, for your health and future success, you may want to make yourself quit the smoking habit.

Don't Trust the Big-Name Food Companies

I know we like to believe everything we read on the back of a box, but the so-called "Nutrition Facts" derived from our processed food containers are not always being completely truthful with us. We need to do some of our own research. Don't place all of your faith in marketers and advertisers who simply wish for you to spend money. These organizations after all are the same ones that brought us harmful things such as high fructose, GMO's and trans-fat. Don't trust the big-name food companies. And if you think you don't need it; *then don't eat it.*

Use Mindful Eating to Help You Meet Your Goals

It is incredible how much we can benefit simply by practicing a little bit of mindfulness and being aware of where we are and what we are doing when we eat. Instead of thinking about the bills or the pressures at work, we need to focus on the food we are eating. We need to focus on the right here, and the right now. It may sound a little silly at first, but don't let your mind wander and allow yourself to focus on the act of eating itself. That way you can use mindful eating to help you meet your goals.

Conclusion: Paleolithic for Life!

First of all, I would like to give you a little pat on the back for finishing this book. And if you follow the guidelines presented herein I have no doubt in my mind that you will be able to succeed 30 Day Paleo Challenge as well. The recipes and bits of advice found in this book serve to guide you in a direction that leads to improved overall health and stamina. It is not about starving yourself, or counting carbs; the 30-Day Paleo Challenge is more than a diet or any other kind of food regimen. The 30-Day Paleo Challenge is a distinct way of life. Thank you for reading!

Made in the USA
Middletown, DE
18 January 2018